HORMONE RESET DIET FOR WOMEN OVER 40

21 Days Hormone Resetting/Balancing Plan to Boost/Heal Your Metabolism and Lose Weight Quickly for Healthy Living.

Dr. Martins Sant

About The Author

Dr. Martins Sant is not just a name; he's your dedicated partner on the journey to a healthier and happier you. With over a decade of experience as a distinguished Nutritionist and Dietitian, Dr. Sant has helped countless individuals transform their lives through the power of proper nutrition.

Armed with a Master's Degree in Nutrition, Dr. Sant's expertise extends far beyond the classroom. He combines his extensive academic knowledge with a profound passion for wellness to create practical and personalized nutrition plans that bring tangible results.

He is on a mission to empower you with the knowledge and tools to make informed dietary choices that enhance your vitality, longevity, and overall well-being. Dr. Sant understands that every person is unique, and he tailors his guidance to suit your individual needs and goals.

Whether you're looking to shed those extra pounds, manage chronic health conditions, or simply adopt a balanced and nutritious lifestyle, Dr. Martins Sant is your go-to expert. His compassionate and approachable demeanor, coupled with a deep commitment to your success, make him a trusted advisor you can rely on.

Join Dr. Sant on a journey to unlock the secrets of nourishing your body and achieving the best version of yourself. With his guidance, you'll discover that optimal health is within your reach, and a fulfilling, nutritious life is just a choice away.

TABLE OF CONTENTS

INTRODUCTION

Hormonal Imbalances in Women Over 40

Hormonal imbalances in women over 40 represent a critical and often overlooked aspect of women's health. As women age, their bodies undergo significant changes, many of which are hormonally driven. Understanding these changes is crucial for maintaining health and well-being during midlife and beyond. This introduction aims to explore the nature of these hormonal changes, their impacts, and the broader context in which they occur.

Understanding Hormonal Changes in Women Over 40

Around the age of 40, women typically experience shifts in their hormonal balance, a prelude to the more widely recognized phase of menopause. This period, often referred to as perimenopause, is marked by fluctuations in the levels of key hormones, primarily estrogen and progesterone. These fluctuations can vary greatly from one woman to another in both intensity and duration.

Estrogen and progesterone are the primary female sex hormones responsible for regulating the menstrual cycle and playing a vital role in maintaining overall health. Estrogen, for example, has protective effects on bone density and heart health, while progesterone helps to prepare the uterus for pregnancy and affects mood regulation.

As women approach their late 40s and early 50s, the ovaries gradually reduce their production of these hormones, leading to perimenopause and eventually menopause. This transition is not sudden but a gradual process that can last several years.

Physical and Emotional Impacts of Hormonal Changes

The consequences of these hormonal fluctuations are both physical and emotional. Common physical symptoms include hot flashes, night sweats, irregular periods, weight gain (especially around the abdomen), thinning hair, dry skin, and increased fatigue. These symptoms can be mildly inconvenient for some, but severely debilitating for others.

From an emotional standpoint, the hormonal changes can lead to mood swings, irritability, anxiety, and depression. These emotional symptoms are often exacerbated by the physical discomforts and the psychological impact of aging and the associated life transitions, such as children leaving home or the onset of chronic health issues.

Hormones and Metabolic Changes

One of the most notable impacts of hormonal changes in women over 40 is on metabolism. The decrease in estrogen levels is associated with a lower metabolic rate, making it easier to gain weight and harder to lose it. This metabolic slowdown is often accompanied by changes in body composition, such as an increase in abdominal fat, which is linked to higher risks of heart disease and diabetes.

Additionally, these hormonal changes can affect insulin sensitivity, cholesterol levels, and blood pressure, all of which are critical factors in metabolic health. This underscores the importance of a tailored approach to diet and lifestyle for women in this age group.

Broader Context of Hormonal Changes

It's essential to understand these hormonal changes within a broader life context. Women over 40 often juggle multiple responsibilities, including careers, family care, and social obligations. These stressors can exacerbate hormonal symptoms and impact overall health.

Moreover, societal attitudes towards aging, particularly for women, can influence how these changes are experienced and managed. The stigma associated with menopause and aging can lead to feelings of isolation or embarrassment, preventing women from seeking the help and support they need.

Addressing Hormonal Imbalances

Addressing hormonal imbalances in women over 40 involves a multifaceted approach. It includes lifestyle modifications such as diet and exercise, stress management techniques, and, in some cases, medical interventions like hormone replacement therapy (HRT). The decision to use HRT should be made on an individual basis, considering the potential benefits and risks.

Diet and Exercise

A balanced diet rich in whole foods, lean proteins, healthy fats, and complex carbohydrates can help manage weight and provide the nutrients needed for hormonal balance. Regular physical activity, including both aerobic and strength-training exercises, is essential for maintaining muscle mass, supporting metabolism, and improving mood.

Stress Management

Stress can exacerbate hormonal imbalances, so managing stress is vital. Techniques like mindfulness, meditation, yoga, and deep breathing exercises can be effective. Additionally, hobbies and activities that promote relaxation and enjoyment are crucial for emotional well-being.

Medical Interventions

For some women, medical interventions like hormone replacement therapy (HRT) can alleviate symptoms. However, HRT is not without risks and should be considered carefully in consultation with a healthcare provider.

The Role of Support and Community

Navigating hormonal changes can be challenging, and support from family, friends, and healthcare professionals is invaluable. Joining support groups or online communities can provide a sense of belonging and a platform to share experiences and advice.

CHAPTER 1

THE SCIENCE BEHIND HORMONAL RESET

How Diet Influences Hormonal Health

The connection between diet and hormonal health is profound and multifaceted. Hormones like insulin, estrogen, cortisol, and thyroid hormones are heavily influenced by dietary choices.

Insulin And Diet

Mechanism of Insulin Regulation: Insulin is vital for regulating blood glucose levels. After eating, carbohydrates are broken down into glucose, which enters the bloodstream. Insulin helps cells absorb glucose, reducing blood sugar levels.

Impact of Diet on Insulin Sensitivity: A diet high in refined sugars and simple carbohydrates (like white bread, pastries, and sugary drinks) causes rapid spikes in blood sugar. Over time, this can lead to insulin resistance, where cells become less responsive to insulin. This condition is a precursor to type 2 diabetes and metabolic syndrome.

Dietary Approaches for Insulin Management:

Low-Glycemic Index Foods: These foods cause a slower, more gradual increase in blood sugar, aiding in maintaining insulin sensitivity.

Fiber-Rich Foods: High fiber intake slows carbohydrate absorption, preventing blood sugar spikes.

Healthy Fats and Proteins: These macronutrients have minimal impact on blood sugar and can promote satiety, reducing overall carbohydrate intake.

Estrogen and Progesterone

Hormonal Balance in Women: Estrogen and progesterone are critical for reproductive health, mood, and bone density. The balance between these hormones is delicate and can be influenced by diet.

Dietary Influences:

Phytoestrogens: Found in foods like flaxseeds, soy, and legumes, these plant-based compounds can mimic estrogen in the body. They may be particularly beneficial during menopause, helping to alleviate symptoms like hot flashes.

Impact of Processed Foods and Alcohol: Excessive intake of processed foods and alcohol can disrupt hormonal balance. These items can affect liver function, which is crucial for hormone metabolism and excretion.

Cortisol

Cortisol's Role: Often termed the stress hormone, cortisol regulates various processes throughout the body, including metabolism and the immune response. It's also integral to the body's stress response.

Diet's Role in Cortisol Regulation:

Balanced Blood Sugar: Diets that prevent blood sugar spikes can help regulate cortisol levels. Prolonged blood sugar lows or highs can stress the body, prompting cortisol release.

Nutrients that Modulate Cortisol: Omega-3 fatty acids (found in fish and flaxseeds), magnesium (in leafy greens, nuts, and seeds), and vitamin C (in fruits and vegetables) are known to support the body's stress response and may help in regulating cortisol levels.

Thyroid Hormones

Thyroid Function: Thyroid hormones regulate metabolism, energy, and body temperature. An imbalance in these hormones can lead to various health issues, including hypothyroidism or hyperthyroidism.

Dietary Impact on Thyroid Health:

Essential Nutrients for Thyroid Function: Iodine, selenium, and zinc are crucial for thyroid hormone production and metabolism. A deficiency in these nutrients can impair thyroid function.

Sources of Key Nutrients:

Iodine: Found in seafood, dairy, and iodized salt.

Selenium: Present in Brazil nuts, seafood, and meats.

Zinc: Found in meat, shellfish, legumes, and seeds.

Goitrogens: Certain foods like soy and cruciferous vegetables contain goitrogens, which can interfere with thyroid function. However, their impact is usually minimal unless consumed in very large amounts or if there's an existing iodine deficiency.

The Role of Lifestyle in Hormonal Balance

Lifestyle factors play a significant role in hormonal health. Stress management, physical activity, sleep, and environmental factors all contribute to hormonal balance.

Stress Management

Impact of Chronic Stress: Chronic stress leads to prolonged elevation of hormones like cortisol and adrenaline. This can result in various health issues, including hormonal imbalances, increased risk of heart disease, anxiety, depression, and weight gain.

Meditation and Hormonal Health: Meditation has been shown to reduce cortisol levels, thereby aiding in the regulation of stress responses. It can also enhance overall well-being by improving sleep quality and reducing anxiety.

Yoga's Holistic Benefits: Yoga, combining physical postures, breath control, and meditation, can be particularly beneficial for hormonal balance. It not only reduces stress but also positively affects the endocrine system, helping to balance hormones.

Deep Breathing Exercises: Techniques such as diaphragmatic breathing can activate the body's relaxation response, reducing stress hormone levels and leading to a more balanced hormonal state.

Physical Activity

Exercise and Insulin Sensitivity: Regular physical activity is key in managing insulin levels and increasing insulin sensitivity. This is crucial for metabolic health and can prevent conditions like type 2 diabetes.

Endorphins and Mood Regulation: Exercise stimulates the production of endorphins, hormones that act as natural painkillers and mood elevators. This is especially beneficial for women over 40 who may experience mood swings due to hormonal fluctuations.

Exercise and Menstrual Health: Regular exercise can also help in regulating menstrual cycles and reducing symptoms of menopause like hot flashes and night sweats.

Sleep Quality

Regulation of Melatonin and Growth Hormone: Both melatonin, the sleep hormone, and growth hormone, crucial for tissue repair and muscle growth, are regulated during sleep. Disrupted sleep patterns can lead to imbalances in these hormones.

Sleep Hygiene Practices: Establishing a regular sleep schedule, creating a dark, quiet, and cool sleeping environment, and avoiding screens before bedtime can enhance sleep quality, thereby supporting hormonal balance.

Impact on Overall Hormonal Health: Adequate sleep is essential for the proper functioning of the entire endocrine system. It affects the production of hormones related to appetite, stress, and metabolism.

Environmental Toxins

Endocrine Disruptors in Everyday Products: Many common products contain chemicals that can interfere with hormonal function. These include bisphenol A (BPA) in plastics, parabens in cosmetics, and certain pesticides.

Choosing Safer Alternatives: Opting for BPA-free products, organic produce, and natural beauty products can reduce exposure to these harmful chemicals.

Detoxifying Living Spaces: Implementing changes such as using natural cleaning products and air purifiers can also help in reducing exposure to endocrine-disrupting toxins in the environment.

CHAPTER 2

PREPARING FOR YOUR HORMONE RESET JOURNEY

Mental and Emotional Readiness

Understanding the Emotional Impact: Embarking on a hormone reset diet can be an emotional journey. It's not uncommon to experience a range of emotions, from excitement and hope to anxiety and doubt. The first step in preparing mentally and emotionally is to acknowledge these feelings. Understanding that it's normal to feel apprehensive about changing long-held eating habits or worried about the diet's effectiveness can help in managing these emotions.

Cultivating a Positive Mindset: A positive mindset is crucial. This involves shifting focus from what you might be giving up (like sugar or caffeine) to what you'll gain, such as improved energy, better sleep, or hormonal balance. Celebrating small victories, like resisting a sugar craving or trying a new healthy recipe, can boost morale and reinforce a positive attitude.

Stress Management Techniques: Stress can adversely affect hormonal balance. It's important to incorporate stress management techniques into your daily routine. This might include mindfulness practices, yoga, meditation, or simply taking time each day to do something you enjoy. Managing stress is not only beneficial for your hormonal health but also for your overall well-being.

Seeking Support: Embarking on a hormone reset journey can be challenging, and having a support system can make a significant difference. This support could come from friends, family, a healthcare professional, or online communities. Sharing your experiences, challenges, and successes with others who understand can be incredibly validating and motivating.

Setting Realistic Goals and Expectations

Understanding Hormonal Changes: Women over 40 experience natural hormonal fluctuations. Understanding these changes is key to setting realistic goals. For instance, weight loss might be slower than it was in your twenties or thirties due to a slower metabolism. Recognizing and accepting these changes can help in setting goals that are achievable and healthy.

Defining Clear, Achievable Goals: Goals should be specific, measurable, achievable, relevant, and time-bound (SMART). Instead of a vague goal like "improve hormone health," a SMART goal would be "reduce caffeine intake to one cup per day over the next month to improve sleep quality." This approach makes it easier to track progress and stay motivated.

Pacing the Journey: It's important to pace yourself. Making too many changes at once can be overwhelming and unsustainable. Start with one or two changes, such as eliminating sugar or incorporating more vegetables into your diet, and gradually build from there. This gradual approach helps to form lasting habits.

Expecting and Embracing Fluctuations: It's normal to have good days and bad days. Hormone levels can fluctuate due to various factors like stress, sleep patterns, and exercise. Understanding that these fluctuations are part of the journey can help in managing expectations and avoiding discouragement.

Evaluating Progress Beyond the Scale: While weight might be a metric for some, it shouldn't be the only measure of success. Improvements in energy levels, mood, sleep quality, and overall well-being are equally significant indicators of progress. Celebrating these non-scale victories can provide a more comprehensive view of the benefits of the hormone reset diet.

CHAPTER 3

THE SEVEN HORMONAL RESETS

Going Meatless: Benefits and Challenges

Nutritional Considerations for a Plant-Based Approach

1. Protein Sources: One of the primary concerns when eliminating meat from the diet is maintaining adequate protein intake. Plant-based proteins like lentils, beans, tofu, tempeh, and quinoa are excellent alternatives. They provide essential amino acids necessary for muscle maintenance, enzyme production, and overall bodily function. It's crucial to vary protein sources to ensure a comprehensive amino acid profile.

2. Iron Absorption: Iron is vital for oxygen transport and energy production. Plant-based iron, known as non-heme iron, is less easily absorbed by the body compared to heme iron found in meat. Including vitamin C-rich foods (like citrus fruits and bell peppers) in meals can enhance iron absorption. Women over 40, particularly those experiencing perimenopause or menopause, should monitor their iron levels to prevent deficiency.

3. Calcium and Bone Health: With age, maintaining bone health becomes increasingly important. Dairy products are a common source of calcium, but there are plant-based options like fortified plant milks, leafy greens, and almonds. Ensuring adequate vitamin D intake, either through sunlight exposure or supplements, is also crucial for calcium absorption.

4. B12 and Essential Nutrients: Vitamin B12, primarily found in animal products, is essential for nerve function and the production of DNA and red blood cells. Plant-based eaters should consider fortified foods or supplements to meet their B12 needs. Other nutrients to focus on include omega-3 fatty acids (from flaxseeds, chia seeds, and walnuts) and zinc (from nuts, seeds, and legumes).

Balancing Hormones Without Meat

1. Phytoestrogens and Menopause: Plant-based diets are rich in phytoestrogens, compounds that can mimic estrogen in the body. Foods like soy and flaxseeds contain these compounds and can be particularly beneficial for women over 40 experiencing menopausal symptoms due to declining estrogen levels.

Phytoestrogens can help in moderating hot flashes and other menopausal symptoms.

2. Reduced Inflammation: Meat, especially processed and red meat, can contribute to inflammation in the body. Chronic inflammation is linked to numerous health issues, including hormonal imbalances. A plant-based diet rich in fruits, vegetables, whole grains, and nuts can help reduce inflammation, thereby potentially improving hormonal health.

3. Weight Management: Maintaining a healthy weight is crucial for hormonal balance. Plant-based diets are often lower in calories and higher in fiber, which can aid in weight loss or maintenance. This is particularly important for women over 40, as metabolism tends to slow down with age, making weight management more challenging.

4. Gut Health: The gut plays a significant role in hormone regulation. A diet rich in diverse plant foods can promote a healthy gut microbiome. Fiber from plants aids in digestion and helps maintain steady blood sugar levels, which is important for hormonal balance, particularly for insulin.

Challenges and Overcoming Them

1. Social and Cultural Adaptations: Shifting to a meatless diet can be challenging in social settings and cultures where meat is a central part of meals. Finding plant-based options at social gatherings or restaurants, and dealing with questions or criticisms from others, can be daunting.

2. Education and Meal Planning: Successfully maintaining a balanced plant-based diet requires education and planning. Understanding nutritional needs and how to meet them with plant-based foods is essential. Meal planning and preparation become crucial to ensure a diverse and nutritious diet.

3. Managing Cravings and Transition: For those used to having meat in their diet, cravings can be a challenge. Gradually reducing meat intake and finding satisfying plant-based alternatives can ease the transition.

4. Monitoring Health Parameters: Particularly for women over 40, it's important to regularly monitor health parameters like iron levels, B12, calcium, and overall nutritional status to ensure that the dietary shift isn't leading to deficiencies.

Sugar Free: Cutting Out the Sweet Culprit

Understanding Sugar's Impact on Hormones

Sugar, in its simplest form, is a carbohydrate. When consumed, it breaks down into glucose, which is a primary energy source for the body. However, the way sugar impacts hormones goes beyond its role as an energy provider.

Insulin Response: The most direct effect of sugar on hormones is through insulin, a hormone produced by the pancreas. When we consume sugar, our blood glucose levels rise, triggering the pancreas to release insulin. Insulin's job is to facilitate the entry of glucose into cells, where it's used for energy. However, excessive sugar intake can lead to frequent and substantial spikes in insulin.

Insulin Resistance and Diabetes: Over time, high sugar intake can lead to a condition called insulin resistance. This occurs when cells in the body become less responsive to insulin. As a result, the pancreas has to produce more insulin to achieve the same effect, which can strain the pancreas and eventually lead to type 2 diabetes.

Impact on Other Hormones: Sugar doesn't just affect insulin. It also influences other hormones, including leptin and ghrelin, which regulate appetite and satiety. High sugar consumption can disrupt the balance between these hormones, leading to increased hunger, overeating, and weight gain.

Stress Hormones: Sugar can also impact stress hormones like cortisol. Fluctuating blood sugar levels can trigger the body's stress response, leading to increased cortisol production. Chronic high cortisol can disrupt sleep, mood, and further exacerbate insulin resistance.

The Role of Sugar in Hormonal Imbalances in Women Over 40

As women age, particularly during and after the menopause transition, hormonal fluctuations become more pronounced. Estrogen and progesterone levels change, which can make the body more sensitive to the effects of sugar.

Menopause and Insulin Sensitivity: The decline in estrogen during menopause can lead to decreased insulin sensitivity and increased abdominal fat. This makes managing sugar intake even more crucial for women over 40.

Impact on Mood and Energy: Fluctuating blood sugar levels can lead to mood swings and energy crashes. This is particularly relevant for women over 40, who may already be experiencing mood fluctuations due to hormonal changes.

Strategies to Manage Sugar Intake

Managing sugar intake is not just about cutting back on sweets; it involves understanding and modifying one's overall dietary habits.

Identifying Hidden Sugars: Sugar is present in many foods, often hidden under various names like fructose, dextrose, or high-fructose corn syrup. Reading labels and being aware of hidden sugars in processed foods is crucial.

Balancing the Diet: A balanced diet that includes a mix of proteins, fats, and complex carbohydrates can help stabilize blood sugar levels. This means opting for whole grains, vegetables, and healthy fats over refined carbs and sugary snacks.

Mindful Eating: Being mindful of when and why you're reaching for sugary foods can also help. Often, sugar cravings are driven by emotional factors like stress or boredom. Recognizing these triggers can lead to healthier coping mechanisms.

Natural Sweeteners and Moderation: Using natural sweeteners like stevia or honey in moderation can be a way to satisfy sweet cravings without the same hormonal impact as refined sugar. However, moderation is key, as overconsumption of any sweetener can lead to similar issues.

Regular Exercise: Exercise is another critical factor in managing blood sugar levels. Regular physical activity improves insulin sensitivity and helps regulate blood sugar.

Healthy Alternatives and Sweetener Options

Sugar, particularly in its refined form, is known to have several adverse effects on health. It can lead to spikes in blood sugar levels, contribute to weight gain, and even affect hormone balance. For women over 40, who are often dealing with hormonal shifts, reducing sugar intake can be crucial for maintaining health and wellness.

Natural Sweeteners: A Healthier Choice

Replacing refined sugar with natural sweeteners can be a healthier option. Natural sweeteners are derived from plants or other natural sources and often undergo less processing than refined sugar. Some popular natural sweeteners include:

Stevia: Derived from the leaves of the stevia plant, it is much sweeter than sugar but has no calories. Stevia does not raise blood sugar levels, making it a good choice for people with diabetes or those looking to control their blood sugar.

Honey: While honey does contain sugar, it also offers additional nutrients like antioxidants. It has a lower glycemic index than sugar, meaning it doesn't spike blood sugar levels as much. Raw, unprocessed honey is the healthiest choice.

Maple Syrup: Made from the sap of maple trees, it contains antioxidants and minerals like manganese and zinc. Maple syrup has a lower glycemic index compared to sugar but is still high in calories and should be used in moderation.

Agave Nectar: Agave nectar comes from the agave plant and is sweeter than sugar, so you can use less of it. However, it's high in fructose, which means it should be used sparingly, especially for those watching their fructose intake.

Dates: Dates can be used to sweeten foods naturally. They are high in fiber, vitamins, and minerals. Dates can be blended into a paste and used in baking or smoothies.

Artificial Sweeteners: Proceed with Caution

Artificial sweeteners like aspartame, sucralose, and saccharin are calorie-free alternatives to sugar. They are much sweeter than sugar, so only a small amount is needed to achieve the same level of sweetness. However, their impact on health and hormone balance is still debated. Some studies suggest they may negatively affect gut health and even lead to cravings for more sugary foods.

Sugar Alcohols: A Middle Ground

Sugar alcohols, such as xylitol, erythritol, and sorbitol, are another alternative. They are lower in calories than sugar and have a lesser impact on blood sugar levels. However, they can cause digestive issues in some people, especially when consumed in large amounts.

Tips for Using Sweeteners

When incorporating these sweeteners into your diet, here are some tips to consider:

Moderation is Key: Even with healthier alternatives, moderation is crucial. Overconsumption of any sweetener can lead to health issues.

Read Labels Carefully: Many products labeled as "sugar-free" or "low sugar" might contain artificial sweeteners or sugar alcohols. It's important to read labels to understand what you're consuming.

Be Mindful of Total Sugar Intake: Remember that natural sweeteners like honey and maple syrup still contribute to your total sugar intake. It's essential to keep track of how much you're using.

Experiment with Reduction: Gradually reducing the amount of sweetener you use can help your palate adjust to less sweetness over time.

Cooking and Baking Adjustments: When substituting sweeteners in recipes, adjustments might be needed. For example, using a liquid sweetener like honey in place of granulated sugar can affect the moisture content of a recipe.

Focus on Whole Foods: Incorporating whole foods like fruits, which provide natural sweetness along with fiber and nutrients, is a healthy approach.

Fruitless: Managing Fructose Intake

The Role of Fruit Sugars in Hormonal Health

Fructose, a natural sugar found in fruits, has a distinct metabolic pathway compared to other sugars like glucose. Unlike glucose, fructose is primarily metabolized in the liver. This unique metabolic process has significant implications for hormonal health, especially in women over 40, who may be experiencing shifts in metabolic efficiency and hormonal balance.

Impact on Insulin and Blood Sugar: Fructose does not stimulate insulin secretion directly, as glucose does. However, a high intake of fructose can lead to insulin resistance over time. Insulin resistance is a condition where the body's cells become less responsive to insulin, leading to higher blood sugar levels and increased insulin production. This imbalance can exacerbate hormonal fluctuations in women over 40, potentially worsening symptoms of menopause and increasing the risk of type 2 diabetes.

Effect on Appetite Regulation: Fructose consumption affects the hormones that regulate appetite, like leptin and ghrelin. Unlike glucose, fructose does not effectively suppress ghrelin, the hunger hormone, and may not stimulate leptin, the satiety hormone, as efficiently. This can lead to an increased caloric intake and weight gain, further impacting hormonal balance.

Liver Health and Fat Storage: Excessive fructose intake is linked to non-alcoholic fatty liver disease (NAFLD), a condition where fat accumulates in the liver. NAFLD can disrupt liver function, affecting the liver's ability to regulate hormones and detoxify the body. Moreover, fructose is more readily converted into fat compared to other sugars, contributing to visceral fat accumulation, which is hormonally active and can disrupt hormonal balance.

Choosing Low-Fructose Options

Given the potential negative impact of high fructose consumption on hormonal health, it's crucial to manage fructose intake. This doesn't mean eliminating fruits altogether, as they are a vital source of vitamins, minerals, and fiber. Instead, the focus should be on selecting low-fructose fruits and balancing fruit consumption with other nutrients.

Selecting Low-Fructose Fruits: Some fruits have lower fructose content and are thus more suitable for a hormone reset diet. These include berries (strawberries, blueberries, raspberries), citrus fruits (oranges, grapefruits), and stone fruits (peaches, plums). These fruits provide the benefits of vitamins, antioxidants, and fiber while minimizing fructose intake.

Portion Control and Timing: Controlling portion sizes and consuming fruits during certain times can help manage fructose intake. Eating fruits with a source of protein or healthy fat can slow down sugar absorption and reduce spikes in blood sugar. For instance, pairing an apple with a handful of almonds can balance the sugar content with healthy fats and protein.

Alternatives to High-Fructose Fruits: For those used to high-fructose fruits like bananas, grapes, and mangoes, transitioning to lower-fructose alternatives can be challenging. Incorporating a variety of low-fructose fruits and experimenting with different recipes can make this transition easier. Smoothies, salads, and fruit-infused water are great ways to enjoy these fruits.

Awareness of Fructose in Processed Foods: It's not just natural fructose in fruits that needs to be managed; many processed foods contain high levels of added fructose, often in the form of high-fructose corn syrup. Reading labels and choosing whole, unprocessed foods can significantly reduce overall fructose intake.

Caffeine Free: Reducing Reliance on Stimulants

How Caffeine Affects Hormonal Balance

Caffeine, a central nervous system stimulant, is widely consumed in various forms such as coffee, tea, and energy drinks. While it's known for its immediate effects like increased alertness and reduced fatigue, caffeine also exerts a less visible but profound impact on the body's hormonal systems.

- **Adrenal Function and Stress Response:** Caffeine stimulates the adrenal glands, leading to increased secretion of stress hormones like cortisol and adrenaline. Over time, this can lead to a state of adrenal fatigue, where the body's response to stress is diminished, and overall energy levels are reduced. For women over 40, who often experience natural hormonal fluctuations, this additional stress on the adrenal system can exacerbate symptoms like fatigue and mood swings.

- **Impact on Estrogen and Other Hormones:** Studies have shown that caffeine can influence the levels of certain hormones, including estrogen. While the effects vary depending on individual factors like genetics and the amount of caffeine consumed, it's clear that caffeine can interact with the hormonal milieu in complex ways. For women in their 40s, particularly those approaching or experiencing menopause, these fluctuations can have significant implications for their hormonal health.

- **Sleep and Melatonin:** Caffeine can disrupt sleep patterns by inhibiting the production of melatonin, the hormone responsible for regulating sleep-wake cycles. Poor sleep quality and insomnia can lead to a cascade of hormonal imbalances, exacerbating issues like weight gain, mood disorders, and decreased immune function.

Transitioning to a Caffeine-Free Life

Making the shift to a caffeine-free lifestyle involves more than just eliminating coffee or tea from your diet. It's a holistic change that embraces alternative methods of managing energy and stress, and requires both physical and psychological adjustments.

- **Gradual Reduction:** To avoid withdrawal symptoms such as headaches, irritability, and fatigue, it's advisable to gradually reduce caffeine intake. This can be done by slowly decreasing the number of caffeinated beverages consumed each day or by switching to lower-caffeine options before completely eliminating caffeine.

- **Alternative Beverages:** Replacing caffeinated drinks with caffeine-free alternatives is crucial. Herbal teas, decaffeinated coffee, and warm water with lemon are healthy options that can satisfy the ritual of a warm drink without the stimulating effects of caffeine.

- **Managing Energy Levels Naturally:** One of the primary reasons people consume caffeine is to boost energy levels. Without caffeine, it's important to find natural ways to maintain energy. Regular physical activity, a balanced diet rich in whole foods, staying hydrated, and ensuring adequate sleep are all critical in this regard.

- Since caffeine is often used as a coping mechanism for stress, finding alternative stress management techniques is vital. Practices such as yoga, meditation, deep breathing exercises, and mindfulness can be highly effective in managing stress without relying on stimulants.

- **Support and Patience:** Transitioning away from caffeine is a journey that requires time and support. Engaging with a community of others who are also reducing caffeine, seeking guidance from healthcare professionals, and being patient with oneself during this transition are essential for success.

Grains and Their Effect on Hormonal Health

The Influence of Grains on Hormones

Grains, a staple in many diets, are rich in carbohydrates. When digested, these carbohydrates break down into sugars, which can influence insulin levels, a key hormone in regulating blood sugar. For women over 40, who may be more susceptible to insulin resistance, this can be particularly impactful. Insulin resistance can disrupt the delicate balance of hormones, potentially leading to conditions such as polycystic ovary syndrome (PCOS), weight gain, and increased risk of type 2 diabetes.

Additionally, certain grains contain gluten, a protein that can trigger inflammatory responses in some individuals. Chronic inflammation can disrupt hormonal activity, leading to imbalances. This is particularly relevant for those with autoimmune conditions like thyroid disorders, which are more common in women as they age.

The Role of Fiber and Nutrients in Grains

Conversely, it's important to recognize the benefits grains can offer. Many are high in fiber, which aids in digestion and can help regulate hormones like estrogen. They also contain various vitamins and minerals essential for hormonal health, such as B vitamins and magnesium. Thus, the decision to eliminate grains should be carefully considered and balanced with the need for these nutrients.

Dairy Free: Understanding Dairy and Hormones

The Link Between Dairy Products and Hormonal Imbalances

- **Biological Impact of Dairy:** Dairy products come from lactating mammals, and thus, inherently contain hormones and growth factors. These substances, while natural to the animals, may not align with human hormonal systems. The primary concern is the presence of insulin-like growth factor-1 (IGF-1), estrogen, and progesterone, which, when introduced into the human body, can potentially disrupt the delicate hormonal balance.

- **Hormonal Sensitivity in Women Over 40:** As women age, particularly during and after their 40s, their bodies undergo significant hormonal changes. Menopause, in particular, marks a drastic shift in hormonal production, primarily estrogen and progesterone. Adding external hormones through diet can exacerbate symptoms like mood swings, weight gain, and even contribute to more severe conditions like osteoporosis or breast cancer.

- **Dairy and Its Systemic Effects:** Research indicates that dairy can influence various hormonal pathways. For instance, dairy's high levels of IGF-1 may promote cell growth, which is a concern in the context of cancer. Additionally, the estrogen in dairy might contribute to estrogen dominance, a condition where the balance of estrogen to progesterone is disrupted, leading to a range of health issues.

- **Individual Responses to Dairy:** It's crucial to acknowledge the variability in how individuals process dairy. Some women may find that dairy exacerbates their hormonal imbalances, while others may not notice significant effects. This variability can be attributed to factors like genetic predisposition, overall diet, lifestyle, and the type of dairy consumed.

Dairy Alternatives for a Balanced Diet

- **Understanding Nutritional Needs:** Eliminating dairy from one's diet necessitates a careful consideration of nutritional replacements. Dairy is a primary source of calcium, vitamin D, and protein for many people. Ensuring these nutrients are adequately supplied through other means is vital for maintaining bone health, muscle function, and overall wellbeing.

- **Plant-Based Milk Alternatives:** Almond, soy, oat, and rice milk are popular dairy substitutes. Each comes with its unique nutritional profile. For example, soy milk is rich in protein, while almond milk offers a good dose of vitamin E. Choosing fortified versions of these milks ensures that you are not missing out on calcium and vitamin D.

- **Calcium-Rich Foods:** Beyond milk substitutes, other foods can provide the necessary calcium.

Leafy green vegetables like kale and broccoli, and fortified foods like certain cereals and juices, are excellent sources. Additionally, nuts, seeds, and legumes also contribute to calcium intake.

- **Protein Sources:** With dairy out of the diet, other protein sources become crucial. Plant-based proteins like lentils, chickpeas, and quinoa, as well as animal-based options like fish, poultry, and eggs, can fill this gap.

- **Vitamin D and Other Nutrients:** Sunlight is a natural source of vitamin D, but for those with limited exposure, supplements may be necessary. Foods like fatty fish, liver, and egg yolks also provide vitamin D. Moreover, ensuring a balanced intake of other nutrients like magnesium and phosphorus is essential for holistic health.

- **Personalized Nutrition:** It's important to tailor dietary choices to individual health needs and preferences. Consulting with a dietitian or nutritionist can provide personalized guidance, ensuring that nutritional needs are met while adhering to a dairy-free diet.

Toxin Free: Purging Harmful Substances

Identifying and Avoiding Endocrine Disruptors

Endocrine Disruptors: A Hidden Threat

Endocrine disruptors are chemicals that can interfere with the endocrine (hormone) system in mammals. These substances can mimic or hinder the actions of hormones, leading to a disruption in the body's normal functions. They are particularly concerning for women over 40, as they can exacerbate or contribute to hormonal imbalances during perimenopause and menopause.

Common Sources of Endocrine Disruptors

Plastics: Substances like Bisphenol A (BPA) and phthalates, often found in plastic bottles and containers, are known endocrine disruptors.

Cosmetics and Personal Care Products: Parabens and certain fragrances used in these products can act as disruptors.

Household Cleaners: Certain chemicals used in these products can be harmful.

Pesticides: Common in agriculture, these chemicals can find their way into our diet.

Industrial Chemicals: Polychlorinated biphenyls (PCBs) and dioxins, though banned or restricted, can still be present in the environment.

Strategies for Avoidance

Opt for Glass or Stainless Steel: When it comes to food and beverage storage, prefer glass or stainless steel over plastic.

Choose Natural Beauty Products: Look for cosmetics and personal care items that are free from parabens and synthetic fragrances.

Use Eco-Friendly Cleaners: Select household cleaning products made with natural ingredients.

Eat Organic: Consuming organic food reduces exposure to pesticides.

Be Informed: Stay updated about potentially harmful chemicals and their sources.

Detoxifying Your Diet and Environment

Detoxifying Your Diet

The idea of detoxifying the diet revolves around minimizing the intake of harmful substances and increasing the consumption of foods that support the body's natural detoxification processes.

Minimize Processed Foods: Highly processed foods often contain additives, preservatives, and other chemicals that can be harmful.

Increase Fiber Intake: Fiber aids in digestion and helps in the elimination of toxins.

Hydration: Water is essential for detoxification, helping to flush out toxins through the kidneys.

Antioxidant-Rich Foods: Foods rich in antioxidants can help protect the body from oxidative stress caused by toxins.

Supportive Supplements: Certain supplements, like milk thistle or turmeric, can support liver health, a crucial organ for detoxification.

Detoxifying Your Environment

Our surroundings can be a significant source of toxins. Reducing exposure in the environment is as crucial as detoxifying the diet.

Air Quality: Use air purifiers, especially in urban settings, and keep indoor plants that can help purify the air.

Clean Water: Consider water filters to remove potential contaminants from tap water.

Natural Cleaning Products: Switch to cleaning products made with natural ingredients.

Mindful Renovation: When renovating, choose materials with low volatile organic compounds (VOCs).

Reduce Electronic Waste: Electronic devices can emit harmful substances; reduce usage and dispose of them responsibly.

CHAPTER 4

REENTRY AND BEYOND

Reentry: Integrating Changes into Everyday Life

Transitioning Back to a Varied Diet

Understanding the Transition Phase: After a period of restrictive eating, reintroducing a wider variety of foods must be approached thoughtfully. The body's response to previously eliminated food groups can vary, and it's important to monitor how you feel during this phase. A gradual reintroduction helps in identifying any food sensitivities or hormonal imbalances that might reoccur.

Step-by-Step Reintroduction: Begin by slowly incorporating one food group at a time, starting with those least likely to disrupt hormonal balance. Whole grains or dairy substitutes can be a good starting point. Maintain a food diary to track your body's reactions, both physically and emotionally, to these reintroduced foods.

Balancing Macronutrients: A balanced diet should include an appropriate mix of carbohydrates, proteins, and fats. Focus on high-fiber carbohydrates like fruits and vegetables, lean proteins, and healthy fats such as avocados and nuts. This balance is crucial in maintaining energy levels and hormonal balance.

Listening to Your Body: Pay attention to signals from your body. Symptoms like bloating, fatigue, or mood swings can indicate a negative response to certain foods. Trusting and understanding your body's cues is vital in maintaining a diet that supports hormonal health.

Maintaining Hormonal Balance Post-Reset

Continued Attention to Diet: Even after the reset diet, certain foods known to disrupt hormonal balance should be consumed in moderation. These include high-sugar foods, refined carbs, and excessive caffeine. Prioritize whole, unprocessed foods to maintain the benefits of the reset.

Regular Physical Activity: Exercise plays a significant role in hormonal balance. Activities like yoga, walking, and strength training can help reduce stress hormones like cortisol and boost endorphins, improving overall hormonal health.

Stress Management Techniques: Chronic stress can significantly impact hormonal balance. Integrating stress-reduction techniques such as meditation, deep breathing exercises, or even engaging in hobbies can help maintain hormonal equilibrium.

Sleep Hygiene: Adequate and quality sleep is essential for hormonal balance. Establish a regular sleep schedule, create a relaxing bedtime routine, and ensure your sleeping environment promotes restfulness.

Regular Health Check-Ups: Regular consultations with healthcare professionals can help monitor hormonal levels and overall health. This is especially important as the body undergoes changes due to age or lifestyle adjustments.

Support Networks: Building a community or joining groups of like-minded individuals who are also focusing on hormonal health can provide motivation and support. Sharing experiences, challenges, and successes can be incredibly encouraging.

Holistic Approach: Remember, hormonal health is not just about diet. It encompasses a holistic approach involving physical, emotional, and mental well-being. Integrating mindful practices, nurturing relationships, and pursuing activities that bring joy are all part of maintaining a healthy hormonal balance.

Sustenance: Long-Term Hormonal Health Strategies

Lifestyle Modifications for Sustained Hormonal Balance

Dietary Adjustments: Post hormone reset, it's vital to continue with a balanced diet that supports hormonal health. This means a diet rich in whole foods, lean proteins, healthy fats, and fiber. Women should focus on including phytoestrogen-rich foods like flaxseeds and soy, which can help in balancing estrogen levels. Cruciferous vegetables like broccoli and cauliflower are also important as they help in the detoxification of excess hormones.

Sleep Quality: Adequate and quality sleep is a cornerstone of hormonal balance. Poor sleep can disrupt the body's natural hormone production, including cortisol and insulin. Women should aim for 7-9 hours of uninterrupted sleep per night. Creating a sleep-conducive environment, maintaining a consistent sleep schedule, and practicing relaxing bedtime rituals can greatly improve sleep quality.

Mindful Eating: Being mindful about eating involves paying attention to hunger and fullness cues, eating slowly, and enjoying meals without distractions. This approach not only improves digestion but also helps in maintaining a healthy weight, which is crucial for hormonal balance.

Avoiding Endocrine Disruptors: Women should continue to be mindful of their exposure to endocrine disruptors found in plastics, certain cosmetics, and household cleaning products. Opting for natural, organic products and reducing plastic use can help in minimizing these exposures.

Stress Management and Physical Activity

Stress Reduction Techniques: Chronic stress can wreak havoc on hormonal balance. Techniques like meditation, yoga, deep breathing exercises, and mindfulness can be effective in managing stress. These practices not only reduce the stress hormone cortisol but also improve overall well-being.

Regular Physical Activity: Exercise is pivotal for hormonal health. It helps in regulating hormones like insulin, improves metabolism, and enhances mood through the release of endorphins. A combination of cardiovascular exercises, strength training, and flexibility workouts is ideal. Activities like brisk walking, swimming, yoga, and weight training can be particularly beneficial for women over 40.

Balancing Exercise and Rest: While regular exercise is crucial, so is rest. Over-exercising can lead to hormonal imbalances due to the stress it places on the body. Listening to the body and including rest days in the exercise regimen is essential.

Holistic Therapies: Holistic therapies such as acupuncture, massage therapy, and reflexology can also support hormonal balance. These therapies can help reduce stress, improve circulation, and enhance the body's natural healing processes.

Social Connections: Maintaining strong social connections and having a support system can greatly impact stress levels and overall health. Engaging in community activities, spending time with loved ones, and pursuing hobbies can provide emotional support and reduce feelings of stress and isolation.

57

CHAPTER 5

RECIPES AND MEAL PLANS

Meatless Phase:

1. Quinoa and Black Bean Stuffed Peppers

Ingredients:

4 large bell peppers, halved and seeded

1 cup cooked quinoa

1 can black beans, drained and rinsed

1/2 cup corn kernels

1/2 cup diced tomatoes

1/4 cup chopped cilantro

1 teaspoon cumin

1/2 teaspoon garlic powder

Salt and pepper to taste

1/2 cup shredded cheese (optional)

Instructions:

Preheat oven to 375°F (190°C).

In a bowl, mix together quinoa, black beans, corn, tomatoes, cilantro, cumin, garlic powder, salt, and pepper.

Stuff each bell pepper half with the quinoa mixture.

Place stuffed peppers in a baking dish and cover with foil.

Bake for 25-30 minutes, or until peppers are tender.

Remove foil, add cheese on top (if using), and bake for an additional 5 minutes or until cheese is melted.

Serve warm.

Nutritional Information:

Calories: 220

Protein: 9g

Carbohydrates: 35g

Fat: 4g

Fiber: 7g

2. Lentil and Vegetable Soup

Ingredients:

1 cup dried lentils, rinsed

1 tablespoon olive oil

1 onion, chopped

2 carrots, diced

2 celery stalks, diced

3 garlic cloves, minced

1 can diced tomatoes

4 cups vegetable broth

1 teaspoon thyme

Salt and pepper to taste

2 cups spinach, chopped

Instructions:

Heat olive oil in a large pot over medium heat.

Add onion, carrots, and celery, and cook until softened.

Stir in garlic and cook for an additional minute.

Add lentils, diced tomatoes, vegetable broth, thyme, salt, and pepper.

Bring to a boil, then reduce heat and simmer for about 30 minutes, or until lentils are tender.

Stir in spinach and cook until wilted.

Adjust seasoning and serve hot.

Nutritional Information:

Calories: 180

Protein: 11g

Carbohydrates: 30g

Fat: 3g

Fiber: 8g

3. Chickpea and Spinach Curry

Ingredients: 1 can chickpeas, drained and rinsed

1 tablespoon olive oil

1 onion, chopped

2 garlic cloves, minced

1 tablespoon curry powder

1 teaspoon turmeric

1 can coconut milk

2 cups spinach, chopped

Salt to taste

Instructions:

Heat olive oil in a skillet over medium heat.

Add onion and garlic, cooking until softened.

Stir in curry powder and turmeric, cooking for another minute.

Add chickpeas and coconut milk, bringing to a simmer.

Cook for 10 minutes, then add spinach and cook until wilted.

Season with salt and serve with brown rice or naan.

Nutritional Information:

Calories: 260

Protein: 9g

Carbohydrates: 25g

Fat: 15g

Fiber: 6g

4. Tofu and Vegetable Stir-Fry

Ingredients:

1 block firm tofu, pressed and cubed

2 tablespoons soy sauce

1 tablespoon sesame oil

1 red bell pepper, sliced

1 cup broccoli florets

1 carrot, sliced

2 garlic cloves, minced

1 teaspoon grated ginger

1 tablespoon olive oil

Instructions:

Marinate tofu in soy sauce and sesame oil for 15 minutes.

Heat olive oil in a wok or large skillet over high heat.

Add tofu and cook until browned on all sides. Remove and set aside.

In the same wok, add bell pepper, broccoli, carrot, garlic, and ginger. Stir-fry until vegetables are tender-crisp.

Return tofu to the wok, stir to combine, and heat through.

Serve with brown rice or quinoa.

Nutritional Information:

Calories: 200

Protein: 12g

Carbohydrates: 15g

Fat: 10g

Fiber: 3g

5. Avocado and Tomato Salad with Lemon Dressing

Ingredients:

2 ripe avocados, diced

2 tomatoes, diced

1/4 cup red onion, finely chopped

1 tablespoon olive oil

Juice of 1 lemon

Salt and pepper to taste

2 tablespoons chopped fresh basil

Instructions:

In a bowl, combine diced avocado, tomato, and red onion.

In a small bowl, whisk together olive oil, lemon juice, salt, and pepper.

Pour dressing over the salad and gently toss to combine.

Garnish with fresh basil and serve immediately.

Nutritional Information:

Calories: 250

Protein: 3g

Carbohydrates: 15g

Fat: 21g

Fiber: 7g

Sugar Free Phase

1. Avocado and Chicken Salad

Ingredients:

1 medium ripe avocado, diced

1 cup cooked chicken breast, shredded

1/4 cup cherry tomatoes, halved

1/4 cup cucumber, diced

1 tablespoon lemon juice

Salt and pepper to taste

1 tablespoon chopped fresh cilantro

Instructions:

In a medium bowl, combine diced avocado, shredded chicken, cherry tomatoes, and cucumber.

Drizzle with lemon juice and season with salt and pepper.

Gently toss to combine everything evenly.

Garnish with fresh cilantro before serving.

Nutritional Information:

Calories: 290

Protein: 25g

Carbohydrates: 9g

Fat: 17g

Fiber: 6g

2. Almond and Herb-Crusted Salmon

Ingredients:

2 salmon fillets (about 6 oz each)

1/4 cup almond flour

1 tablespoon fresh dill, finely chopped

1 tablespoon fresh parsley, finely chopped

1 teaspoon lemon zest

Salt and pepper to taste

1 tablespoon olive oil

Instructions:

Preheat the oven to 375°F (190°C).

In a small bowl, mix almond flour, dill, parsley, lemon zest, salt, and pepper.

Coat each salmon fillet with the almond herb mixture.

Heat olive oil in a skillet over medium heat and sear the salmon for 2 minutes on each side.

Transfer to the oven and bake for 8-10 minutes or until cooked through.

Nutritional Information:

Calories: 350

Protein: 34g

Carbohydrates: 3g

Fat: 22g

Fiber: 2g

3. Zucchini Noodles with Pesto and Pine Nuts

Ingredients:

2 medium zucchinis, spiralized into noodles

1/4 cup pesto sauce (sugar-free)

2 tablespoons pine nuts, toasted

Salt and pepper to taste

Parmesan cheese, grated (optional)

Instructions: In a large skillet, cook the zucchini noodles over medium heat for 2-3 minutes or until slightly softened.

Stir in pesto sauce and season with salt and pepper.

Cook for another 2 minutes, stirring occasionally.

Serve topped with toasted pine nuts and grated Parmesan cheese (if using).

Nutritional Information:

Calories: 190

Protein: 6g

Carbohydrates: 6g

Fat: 16g

Fiber: 2g

4. Cauliflower Rice Stir-Fry with Vegetables

Ingredients:

2 cups cauliflower rice

1/2 cup red bell pepper, diced

1/2 cup broccoli florets

1/4 cup carrot, julienned

2 tablespoons coconut oil

1 teaspoon garlic, minced

2 tablespoons soy sauce (low sodium, sugar-free)

Salt and pepper to taste

Instructions:

In a large skillet, heat coconut oil over medium heat.

Add garlic, red bell pepper, broccoli, and carrot. Stir-fry for 4-5 minutes.

Add cauliflower rice and soy sauce. Cook for an additional 5-7 minutes or until vegetables are tender and cauliflower rice is cooked through.

Season with salt and pepper to taste and serve hot.

Nutritional Information:

Calories: 120

Protein: 4g

Carbohydrates: 12g

Fat: 7g

Fiber: 4g

5. Spinach and Feta Stuffed Chicken Breast

Ingredients:

2 boneless, skinless chicken breasts

1 cup spinach, chopped

1/4 cup feta cheese, crumbled

1 teaspoon olive oil

Salt and pepper to taste

1 teaspoon dried oregano

Instructions:

Preheat oven to 375°F (190°C).

Make a horizontal slit in each chicken breast to create a pocket.

Stuff each pocket with chopped spinach and crumbled feta cheese.

Season the chicken with salt, pepper, and oregano.

In a skillet, heat olive oil over medium heat and sear the chicken on both sides until golden.

Transfer to the oven and bake for 20-25 minutes or until the chicken is cooked through.

Nutritional Information:

Calories: 300

Protein: 38g

Carbohydrates: 2g

Fat: 15g

Fiber: 1g

6. Balsamic Glazed Brussels Sprouts

Ingredients:

2 cups Brussels sprouts, halved

1 tablespoon olive oil

2 tablespoons balsamic vinegar (sugar-free)

Salt and pepper to taste

1/4 cup walnuts, chopped

Instructions:

In a skillet, heat olive oil over medium heat.

Add Brussels sprouts and cook for 5-7 minutes or until they start to brown.

Add balsamic vinegar and continue cooking for 2-3 minutes until sprouts are glazed.

Season with salt and pepper.

Garnish with chopped walnuts before serving.

Nutritional Information:

Calories: 140

Protein: 5g

Carbohydrates: 10g

Fat: 10g

Fiber: 4g

7. Greek Yogurt Parfait with Nuts and Seeds

Ingredients:

1 cup Greek yogurt (unsweetened, full-fat)

1 tablespoon chia seeds

1 tablespoon flaxseeds

1/4 cup mixed nuts (almonds, walnuts, pecans), chopped

Cinnamon to taste

Instructions:

In a bowl, layer Greek yogurt with chia seeds, flaxseeds, and chopped nuts.

Sprinkle cinnamon on top for flavor.

Serve chilled.

Nutritional Information:

Calories: 250

Protein: 15g

Carbohydrates: 10g

Fat: 17g

Fiber: 5g

Fruitless Phase

1. Avocado & Egg Salad

Ingredients:

2 hard-boiled eggs, chopped

1 ripe avocado, cubed

2 tablespoons of chopped chives

1 tablespoon of lemon juice

Salt and pepper to taste

1 tablespoon of extra virgin olive oil

Instructions: In a bowl, combine the chopped hard-boiled eggs and cubed avocado.

Add the chopped chives and lemon juice, and gently mix.

Season with salt and pepper, and drizzle with olive oil.

Serve chilled, either alone or on a bed of leafy greens.

Nutritional Information:

Calories: 400

Protein: 15g

Carbohydrates: 15g

Fat: 34g

Fiber: 7g

2. Cauliflower Rice Stir-Fry

Ingredients:

2 cups of cauliflower rice

1 cup of mixed bell peppers, thinly sliced

1/2 cup of red onion, diced

1 clove of garlic, minced

1 tablespoon of coconut oil

2 tablespoons of soy sauce (gluten-free if needed)

Salt and pepper to taste

Instructions: Heat coconut oil in a large skillet over medium heat.

Sauté red onion and garlic until fragrant.

Add the mixed bell peppers, and cook until slightly tender.

Stir in the cauliflower rice and soy sauce.

Cook for about 5 minutes, stirring frequently, until the cauliflower is tender.

Season with salt and pepper, and serve hot.

Nutritional Information:

Calories: 180

Protein: 4g

Carbohydrates: 20g

Fat: 10g

Fiber: 5g

3. Almond Flour Pancakes

Ingredients:

1 cup of almond flour

2 large eggs

1/3 cup of almond milk

1 teaspoon of baking powder

1 tablespoon of coconut oil (for cooking)

A pinch of salt

Instructions:

In a mixing bowl, combine almond flour, baking powder, and salt.

Whisk in eggs and almond milk until you have a smooth batter.

Heat a non-stick pan and brush with coconut oil.

Pour batter to form pancakes and cook until bubbles form on the surface, then flip and cook until golden brown.

Serve warm.

Nutritional Information:

Calories: 280

Protein: 12g

Carbohydrates: 10g

Fat: 24g

Fiber: 6g

4. Spinach and Mushroom Frittata

Ingredients:

4 large eggs

2 cups of fresh spinach

1 cup of mushrooms, sliced

1/4 cup of grated Parmesan cheese

1 tablespoon of olive oil

Salt and pepper to taste

Instructions: Preheat the oven to 375°F (190°C).

In a skillet, heat olive oil over medium heat. Sauté mushrooms until tender.

Add spinach and cook until wilted.

In a bowl, beat the eggs, then stir in the cooked vegetables and Parmesan cheese.

Pour the mixture into a greased baking dish.

Bake for 20 minutes or until the frittata is set and lightly golden.

Slice and serve warm.

Nutritional Information:

Calories: 220

Protein: 18g

Carbohydrates: 4g

Fat: 15g

Fiber: 2g

5. Zucchini Noodles with Pesto

Ingredients:

2 medium zucchinis, spiralized

1/2 cup of basil pesto

1/4 cup of cherry tomatoes, halved

2 tablespoons of pine nuts

Salt and pepper to taste

1 tablespoon of olive oil

Instructions:

In a pan, heat the olive oil over medium heat.

Add the spiralized zucchini noodles and cook for 3-4 minutes.

Stir in the basil pesto until the noodles are well-coated.

Add the cherry tomatoes and cook for another minute.

Season with salt and pepper.

Serve hot, garnished with pine nuts.

Nutritional Information:

Calories: 320

Protein: 7g

Carbohydrates: 12g

Fat: 28g

Fiber: 4g

Caffeine-Free Phase:

Avocado and Chickpea Salad

Ingredients:

1 ripe avocado, diced

1 cup canned chickpeas, rinsed and drained

1/2 cup cherry tomatoes, halved

1/4 cup red onion, finely chopped

1 tablespoon olive oil

2 tablespoons lemon juice

Salt and pepper to taste

Fresh cilantro, chopped (optional)

Instructions:

In a mixing bowl, combine the diced avocado, chickpeas, cherry tomatoes, and red onion.

Drizzle with olive oil and lemon juice, then season with salt and pepper.

Gently toss the ingredients to combine.

Garnish with fresh cilantro if desired.

Serve immediately or chill in the refrigerator before serving.

Nutritional Information:

Calories: 300

Protein: 9g

Carbohydrates: 35g

Fat: 15g

Fiber: 10g

Turmeric Ginger Herbal Tea

Ingredients:

1-inch fresh turmeric root, thinly sliced

1-inch fresh ginger root, thinly sliced

4 cups water

1 tablespoon honey (optional)

Lemon slices for garnish

Instructions:

In a saucepan, bring water to a boil.

Add the sliced turmeric and ginger to the boiling water.

Reduce heat and simmer for 10-15 minutes.

Strain the tea into cups.

Stir in honey if desired and garnish with a slice of lemon.

Serve hot.

Nutritional Information:

Calories (without honey): 10

Protein: 0g

Carbohydrates: 2g

Fat: 0g

Fiber: 0g

Kale and Quinoa Superfood Bowl

Ingredients: 1 cup cooked quinoa

2 cups kale, chopped

1/2 cup roasted sweet potato cubes

1/4 cup dried cranberries

1/4 cup chopped walnuts

2 tablespoons balsamic vinaigrette

Instructions:

In a bowl, combine the cooked quinoa, chopped kale, roasted sweet potato cubes, dried cranberries, and chopped walnuts.

Drizzle with balsamic vinaigrette and toss to combine.

Serve immediately or store in the refrigerator for a quick grab-and-go meal.

Nutritional Information:

Calories: 420

Protein: 12g

Carbohydrates: 58g

Fat: 18g

Fiber: 8g

Almond Butter and Banana Smoothie

Ingredients:

1 ripe banana

2 tablespoons almond butter

1 cup unsweetened almond milk

1/2 teaspoon cinnamon

1 tablespoon flaxseeds

Instructions:

In a blender, combine the banana, almond butter, almond milk, cinnamon, and flaxseeds.

Blend until smooth.

Serve immediately in a tall glass.

Nutritional Information:

Calories: 330

Protein: 8g

Carbohydrates: 35g

Fat: 19g

Fiber: 7g

Roasted Cauliflower and Lentil Salad

Ingredients:

2 cups cauliflower florets

1 cup cooked green lentils

1/2 cup arugula

1/4 cup diced red bell pepper

2 tablespoons olive oil

1 tablespoon red wine vinegar

Salt and pepper to taste

1/4 teaspoon smoked paprika

Instructions:

Preheat the oven to 400°F (200°C).

Toss the cauliflower florets with 1 tablespoon olive oil, salt, pepper, and smoked paprika.

Roast in the oven for 20-25 minutes, or until tender and golden.

In a bowl, combine the roasted cauliflower, cooked lentils, arugula, and diced red bell pepper.

Drizzle with the remaining olive oil and red wine vinegar.

Toss to combine and season with additional salt and pepper if needed.

Serve warm or at room temperature.

Nutritional Information:

Calories: 290

Protein: 14g

Carbohydrates: 38g

Fat: 10g

Fiber: 15g

Grain-Free Phase:

1. Avocado and Smoked Salmon Salad

Ingredients:

2 cups mixed greens (spinach, arugula, lettuce)

4 oz smoked salmon, sliced

1 ripe avocado, sliced

1/4 cup cherry tomatoes, halved

1/4 red onion, thinly sliced

2 tablespoons olive oil

1 tablespoon apple cider vinegar

Salt and pepper to taste

1 tablespoon lemon juice

1 teaspoon mustard (Dijon or whole grain)

Instructions:

In a large bowl, combine mixed greens, smoked salmon, avocado slices, cherry tomatoes, and red onion.

In a small bowl, whisk together olive oil, apple cider vinegar, lemon juice, mustard, salt, and pepper to make the dressing.

Drizzle the dressing over the salad and toss gently to combine.

Serve immediately.

Nutritional Information:

Calories: 380

Protein: 23g

Carbohydrates: 12g

Fat: 28g

Fiber: 7g

2. Mediterranean Chicken Skewers

Ingredients:

2 boneless, skinless chicken breasts, cut into chunks

1 zucchini, sliced into rounds

1 bell pepper, cut into chunks

1/2 red onion, cut into chunks

2 tablespoons olive oil

1 teaspoon dried oregano

1 teaspoon garlic powder

Salt and pepper to taste

Lemon wedges for serving

Instructions:

Preheat the grill to medium-high heat.

Thread chicken, zucchini, bell pepper, and red onion alternately onto skewers.

In a small bowl, mix olive oil, oregano, garlic powder, salt, and pepper.

Brush the mixture over the skewers.

Grill skewers, turning occasionally, until the chicken is cooked through, about 10-15 minutes.

Serve with lemon wedges.

Nutritional Information:

Calories: 300

Protein: 26g

Carbohydrates: 8g

Fat: 18g

Fiber: 2g

3. Cauliflower Rice Stir-Fry

Ingredients:

2 cups riced cauliflower

1 cup broccoli florets

1/2 cup carrots, sliced

1/2 cup bell pepper, diced

1/4 cup peas

2 tablespoons coconut oil

1 tablespoon soy sauce or tamari

1 teaspoon ginger, minced

2 cloves garlic, minced

Salt and pepper to taste

Instructions:

Heat coconut oil in a large skillet over medium heat.

Add ginger and garlic, sauté for 1 minute.

Add broccoli, carrots, and bell peppers, cook for 5 minutes.

Stir in riced cauliflower, peas, soy sauce, salt, and pepper.

Cook for another 5-7 minutes until vegetables are tender and cauliflower rice is heated through.

Serve hot.

Nutritional Information:

Calories: 180

Protein: 6g

Carbohydrates: 14g

Fat: 12g

Fiber: 5g

4. Spinach and Mushroom Frittata

Ingredients: 6 large eggs

1 cup fresh spinach, chopped

1/2 cup mushrooms, sliced

1/4 cup red bell pepper, diced

1/4 cup grated Parmesan cheese

2 tablespoons olive oil

Salt and pepper to taste

Instructions:

Preheat oven to 375°F (190°C).

In a bowl, whisk together eggs, Parmesan, salt, and pepper.

Heat olive oil in an oven-proof skillet over medium heat.

Sauté mushrooms and bell pepper until soft.

Add spinach and cook until wilted.

Pour egg mixture over vegetables in the skillet.

Cook for 2-3 minutes until the edges start to set.

Transfer skillet to oven and bake for 8-10 minutes until the frittata is set and golden.

Serve warm.

Nutritional Information:

Calories: 220

Protein: 15g

Carbohydrates: 4g

Fat: 16g

Fiber: 1g

5. Lemon-Garlic Shrimp and Asparagus

Ingredients:

1 lb shrimp, peeled and deveined

2 cups asparagus, trimmed and cut into pieces

3 tablespoons olive oil

2 cloves garlic, minced

Zest and juice of 1 lemon

Salt and pepper to taste

Fresh parsley for garnish

Instructions:

Heat 2 tablespoons of olive oil in a large skillet over medium-high heat.

Add asparagus and cook until tender-crisp, about 3-4 minutes.

Remove asparagus and set aside.

In the same skillet, add the remaining olive oil and garlic.

Add shrimp and cook until pink and opaque, about 2-3 minutes per side.

Return asparagus to the skillet, add lemon zest, lemon juice, salt, and pepper.

Toss to combine and cook for an additional minute.

Garnish with fresh parsley before serving.

Nutritional Information:

Calories: 250

Protein: 24g

Carbohydrates: 6g

Fat: 14g

Fiber: 2g

Avocado and Black Bean Salad

Ingredients:

1 ripe avocado, diced

1 cup cooked black beans

1/2 cup cherry tomatoes, halved

1/4 cup red onion, finely chopped

1/4 cup cilantro, chopped

Juice of 1 lime

Salt and pepper to taste

1 tablespoon olive oil

Instructions:

In a large bowl, combine the diced avocado, cooked black beans, cherry tomatoes, and red onion.

Add chopped cilantro, lime juice, olive oil, salt, and pepper.

Toss gently to combine all ingredients.

Serve chilled or at room temperature.

Nutritional Information:

Calories: 220

Protein: 8g

Carbohydrates: 24g

Fat: 11g

Fiber: 10g

Quinoa and Roasted Vegetable Bowl

Ingredients:

1/2 cup quinoa

1 cup vegetable broth

1 small zucchini, sliced

1 red bell pepper, chopped

1/2 cup cherry tomatoes

1 tablespoon olive oil

Salt and pepper to taste

1 tablespoon balsamic vinegar

Instructions:

Preheat the oven to 400°F (200°C).

Toss zucchini, bell pepper, and cherry tomatoes with olive oil, salt, and pepper.

Roast vegetables in the oven for 20 minutes or until tender.

Mix cooked quinoa with roasted vegetables and drizzle with balsamic vinegar.

Serve warm or at room temperature.

Nutritional Information:

Calories: 320

Protein: 9g

Carbohydrates: 45g

Fat: 12g

Fiber: 6g

Almond Butter and Banana Smoothie

Ingredients:

1 banana

2 tablespoons almond butter

1 cup unsweetened almond milk

1/2 teaspoon vanilla extract

1 tablespoon chia seeds

Ice cubes (optional)

Instructions: Combine banana, almond butter, almond milk, vanilla extract, and chia seeds in a blender.

Add ice cubes if desired for a colder smoothie.

Blend until smooth and creamy.

Serve immediately.

Nutritional Information:

Calories: 300

Protein: 8g

Carbohydrates: 35g

Fat: 16g

Fiber: 7g

Spicy Lentil Soup

Ingredients:

1 cup red lentils, rinsed

1 onion, chopped

2 cloves garlic, minced

1 carrot, chopped

4 cups vegetable broth

1 teaspoon ground cumin

1/2 teaspoon chili powder

Salt and pepper to taste

1 tablespoon olive oil

Instructions:

Heat olive oil in a large pot over medium heat.

Sauté onion, garlic, and carrot until soft.

Add red lentils, vegetable broth, cumin, chili powder, salt, and pepper.

Bring to a boil, then reduce heat and simmer for 20-25 minutes or until lentils are soft.

Serve hot.

Nutritional Information:

Calories: 250

Protein: 15g

Carbohydrates: 35g

Fat: 5g

Fiber: 16g

Stir-Fried Tofu with Broccoli and Peppers

Ingredients:

1 block firm tofu, pressed and cubed

1 head broccoli, cut into florets

1 red bell pepper, sliced

2 tablespoons soy sauce (gluten-free if necessary)

1 tablespoon sesame oil

1 teaspoon ginger, grated

2 cloves garlic, minced

Salt and pepper to taste

1 tablespoon olive oil for cooking

Instructions:

Heat olive oil in a large skillet or wok over medium-high heat.

Add tofu and cook until golden brown on all sides.

Remove tofu and set aside.

In the same skillet, add sesame oil, ginger, garlic, broccoli, and bell pepper. Stir-fry until vegetables are tender but crisp.

Return tofu to the skillet, add soy sauce, and toss everything together.

Season with salt and pepper as needed.

Serve hot.

Nutritional Information:

Calories: 280

Protein: 18g

Carbohydrates: 20g

Fat: 15g

Fiber: 6g

Toxin-Free Phase:

1. Avocado and Walnut Salad

Ingredients:

1 ripe avocado, sliced

1/2 cup walnuts, chopped

2 cups mixed greens (spinach, arugula, and kale)

1/4 cup cherry tomatoes, halved

1/4 cup cucumber, sliced

2 tablespoons extra virgin olive oil

1 tablespoon lemon juice

Salt and pepper to taste

Instructions:

In a large bowl, combine mixed greens, cherry tomatoes, and cucumber slices.

Add the sliced avocado and chopped walnuts to the salad.

In a small bowl, whisk together extra virgin olive oil, lemon juice, salt, and pepper to create a dressing.

Drizzle the dressing over the salad and toss gently to combine.

Serve immediately for a fresh, nutrient-rich meal.

Nutritional Information:

Calories: 380

Protein: 6g

Carbohydrates: 20g

Fat: 34g

Fiber: 8g

2. Quinoa and Roasted Vegetable Bowl

Ingredients:

1 cup quinoa, rinsed

2 cups water

1 cup broccoli florets

1 cup diced sweet potato

1 red bell pepper, sliced

2 tablespoons olive oil

1/2 teaspoon garlic powder

Salt and pepper to taste

1 tablespoon tahini (optional)

Instructions:

Preheat the oven to 400°F (200°C).

Place broccoli, sweet potato, and bell pepper on a baking sheet. Drizzle with olive oil and sprinkle with garlic powder, salt, and pepper. Roast for 20-25 minutes until vegetables are tender.

Meanwhile, bring quinoa and water to a boil in a pot. Reduce heat to low, cover, and simmer for 15 minutes until water is absorbed.

Fluff the cooked quinoa with a fork and divide it among bowls.

Top the quinoa with roasted vegetables. Drizzle with tahini if desired.

Serve warm, enjoying a hearty and nutritious meal.

Nutritional Information:

Calories: 320

Protein: 10g

Carbohydrates: 45g

Fat: 12g

Fiber: 7g

3. Grilled Lemon-Herb Chicken

Ingredients:

2 boneless, skinless chicken breasts

2 tablespoons olive oil

1 lemon, juiced and zested

2 cloves garlic, minced

1 teaspoon dried rosemary

1 teaspoon dried thyme

Salt and pepper to taste

Instructions:

In a bowl, mix olive oil, lemon juice and zest, garlic, rosemary, thyme, salt, and pepper.

Add chicken breasts to the marinade, ensuring they are well coated. Marinate for at least 30 minutes in the refrigerator.

Preheat grill to medium-high heat.

Grill the chicken for 6-8 minutes on each side, until cooked through and juices run clear.

Serve hot, garnished with lemon slices and additional herbs if desired.

Nutritional Information:

Calories: 260

Protein: 35g

Carbohydrates: 3g

Fat: 12g

Fiber: 1g

4. Baked Salmon with Asparagus

Ingredients:

2 salmon fillets (4 oz each)

1 bunch asparagus, trimmed

2 tablespoons olive oil

1 lemon, sliced

Salt and pepper to taste

1 teaspoon dill (optional)

Instructions: Preheat oven to 400°F (200°C).

Place salmon fillets and asparagus on a baking sheet.

Drizzle with olive oil, and season with salt, pepper, and dill.

Top with lemon slices.

Bake for 12-15 minutes, until salmon is cooked through and asparagus is tender.

Serve immediately, enjoying the blend of flavors.

Nutritional Information:

Calories: 300

Protein: 25g

Carbohydrates: 6g

Fat: 20g

Fiber: 3g

5. Berry and Chia Pudding

Ingredients:

1/4 cup chia seeds

1 cup unsweetened almond milk

1 tablespoon honey (optional)

1/2 cup mixed berries (blueberries, raspberries, strawberries)

1 teaspoon vanilla extract

Instructions:

In a bowl, mix chia seeds with almond milk, vanilla extract, and honey if using. Stir well.

Refrigerate for at least 4 hours or overnight until it reaches a pudding-like consistency.

Before serving, top the pudding with mixed berries.

Enjoy a delicious and nutritious dessert or breakfast.

Nutritional Information:

Calories: 200

Protein: 5g

Carbohydrates: 25g

Fat: 10g

Fiber: 10g

Healthy 21 Days Meal Plan

Week 1

Day 1: Meatless

Breakfast: Spinach and Mushroom Omelet (use egg whites if avoiding whole eggs)

Lunch: Quinoa Salad with Roasted Vegetables

Dinner: Grilled Tofu with a Side of Steamed Broccoli and Carrots

Snacks: Almonds; Celery Sticks with Hummus

Day 2: Sugar-Free

Breakfast: Greek Yogurt with Nuts (unsweetened yogurt)

Lunch: Grilled Chicken Salad with Olive Oil and Lemon Dressing

Dinner: Baked Salmon with Asparagus and a Side Salad

Snacks: Cucumber Slices; Hard-Boiled Egg

Day 3: Fruitless

Breakfast: Scrambled Eggs with Spinach and Avocado

Lunch: Lentil Soup with a Side of Mixed Greens

Dinner: Stir-Fried Tofu with Mixed Vegetables (bell peppers, zucchini, etc.)

Snacks: Raw Walnuts; Sliced Bell Peppers

Day 4: Caffeine-Free

Breakfast: Chia Seed Pudding with Almond Milk

Lunch: Turkey Lettuce Wraps with Cucumber and Carrot

Dinner: Baked Cod with Lemon and Dill, Served with Quinoa

Snacks: Pumpkin Seeds; Sliced Cucumber with Guacamole

Day 5: Grain-Free

Breakfast: Veggie Frittata (egg-based, with tomatoes, onions, and bell peppers)

Lunch: Chicken Caesar Salad (without croutons)

Dinner: Grilled Shrimp with a Spinach and Avocado Salad

Snacks: Olives; Sliced Turkey Breast

Day 6: Dairy-Free

Breakfast: Smoothie with Spinach, Almond Milk, and Peanut Butter

Lunch: Chickpea Salad with Olive Oil and Vinegar Dressing

Dinner: Beef Stir-Fry with Cauliflower Rice

Snacks: Roasted Almonds; Carrot Sticks

Day 7: Toxin-Free

Breakfast: Oatmeal with Cinnamon and Almond Milk (ensure gluten-free if necessary)

Lunch: Baked Chicken Breast with Steamed Green Beans

Dinner: Grilled Vegetable Skewers with Herb-Marinated Tofu

Snacks: Sunflower Seeds; Sliced Apples with Almond Butter (assuming toxins refer to artificial additives)

Week 2

Day 1: Meatless

Breakfast: Avocado Toast on Whole Grain Bread (use gluten-free bread if necessary)

Lunch: Lentil and Vegetable Stew

Dinner: Stuffed Bell Peppers with Quinoa and Black Beans

Snacks: Roasted Chickpeas; Baby Carrots

Day 2: Sugar-Free

Breakfast: Omelet with Onions, Peppers, and Spinach

Lunch: Grilled Turkey Breast with a Side of Sautéed Kale

Dinner: Baked White Fish with a Side of Roasted Brussels Sprouts

Snacks: Cucumber Slices; Mixed Nuts

Day 3: Fruitless

Breakfast: Poached Eggs with Sautéed Spinach and Mushrooms

Lunch: Chicken and Vegetable Soup

Dinner: Beef and Vegetable Stir-Fry (using low-sodium soy sauce)

Snacks: Sliced Avocado; Pumpkin Seeds

Day 4: Caffeine-Free

Breakfast: Banana Pancakes made with Almond Flour (use a sugar-free recipe)

Lunch: Tuna Salad with Lettuce and Cherry Tomatoes

Dinner: Roasted Chicken Thighs with Garlic and Herbs, served with Steamed Broccoli

Snacks: Boiled Eggs; Bell Pepper Strips

Day 5: Grain-Free

Breakfast: Smoothie Bowl with Coconut Milk, Spinach, and Chia Seeds

Lunch: Grilled Salmon Salad with Mixed Greens and Olive Oil Dressing

Dinner: Pork Chops with a Side of Roasted Butternut Squash

Snacks: Almond Butter; Celery Sticks

Day 6: Dairy-Free

Breakfast: Scrambled Tofu with Turmeric, Onions, and Tomatoes

Lunch: Quinoa Salad with Cucumber, Tomatoes, and Lemon Vinaigrette

Dinner: Grilled Eggplant and Zucchini with a Side of Chickpeas

Snacks: Sunflower Seeds; Sliced Cucumbers

Day 7: Toxin-Free

Breakfast: Coconut Yogurt with Gluten-Free Granola

Lunch: Baked Lemon-Garlic Tilapia with a Side of Steamed Asparagus

Dinner: Veggie Curry with Cauliflower Rice

Snacks: Homemade Trail Mix (nuts, seeds, unsweetened coconut flakes); Fresh Vegetable Sticks

Week 3

Day 1: Meatless

Breakfast: Greek Yogurt Parfait with Nuts and Seeds (use dairy-free yogurt if preferred)

Lunch: Chickpea Salad with Tomatoes, Cucumbers, and a Lemon-Tahini Dressing

Dinner: Eggplant Parmesan (with dairy-free cheese)

Snacks: Edamame; Sliced Bell Peppers

Day 2: Sugar-Free

Breakfast: Scrambled Eggs with Sautéed Greens and Mushrooms

Lunch: Turkey Lettuce Wraps with Avocado and Sliced Tomato

Dinner: Grilled Pork Loin with a Side of Green Beans Almondine

Snacks: Raw Almonds; Cherry Tomatoes

Day 3: Fruitless

Breakfast: Veggie Omelet with Spinach, Tomatoes, and Onions

Lunch: Beef and Vegetable Soup

Dinner: Baked Lemon-Herb Chicken Breast with Roasted Cauliflower

Snacks: Sliced Cucumbers; Hard-Boiled Eggs

Day 4: Caffeine-Free

Breakfast: Coconut Milk Smoothie with Spinach, Peanut Butter, and Protein Powder

Lunch: Chicken Caesar Salad (without croutons, use a dairy-free dressing)

Dinner: Baked Cod with a Side of Sautéed Zucchini and Squash

Snacks: Walnuts; Sliced Red Pepper

Day 5: Grain-Free

Breakfast: Almond Flour Pancakes with a Berry Compote (sugar-free)

Lunch: Grilled Shrimp over a Mixed Green Salad with Olive Oil and Lemon Dressing

Dinner: Stuffed Peppers with Ground Turkey and Vegetables

Snacks: Guacamole; Sliced Cucumber

Day 6: Dairy-Free

Breakfast: Smoothie with Almond Milk, Kale, Avocado, and Flaxseeds

Lunch: Quinoa and Black Bean Stuffed Sweet Potatoes

Dinner: Stir-Fried Tofu with Mixed Vegetables in a Ginger-Soy Sauce

Snacks: Roasted Pumpkin Seeds; Carrot Sticks

Day 7: Toxin-Free

Breakfast: Oatmeal with Cinnamon and Nutmeg (ensure gluten-free oats)

Lunch: Grilled Chicken Salad with Mixed Greens, Cucumbers, and Carrots

Dinner: Baked Salmon with a Side of Steamed Broccoli and Lemon

Snacks: Sunflower Seeds; Fresh Veggie Sticks

Week 4

Day 1: Meatless

Breakfast: Chia Pudding with Almond Milk and a Sprinkle of Cinnamon

Lunch: Vegetable Stir-Fry with Tofu and a Soy-Ginger Glaze

Dinner: Vegetarian Chili with Kidney Beans, Bell Peppers, and Onions

Snacks: Roasted Seaweed; Sliced Cucumber

Day 2: Sugar-Free

Breakfast: Boiled Eggs with Sautéed Spinach and Tomatoes

Lunch: Grilled Chicken Breast with Mixed Greens and Avocado

Dinner: Baked Trout with Lemon and Dill, Served with Steamed Asparagus

Snacks: Almonds; Cherry Tomatoes

Day 3: Fruitless

Breakfast: Spinach and Feta (dairy-free) Omelet

Lunch: Beef and Vegetable Kebabs

Dinner: Roasted Turkey Breast with Garlic Green Beans

Snacks: Celery Sticks with Almond Butter; Olives

Day 4: Caffeine-Free

Breakfast: Yogurt (dairy-free) with Flaxseeds and Walnut Pieces

Lunch: Tuna Salad with Mixed Greens, Cucumbers, and Olives

Dinner: Lemon-Herbed Chicken Thighs with Roasted Brussel Sprouts

Snacks: Hard-Boiled Eggs; Sliced Bell Peppers

Day 5: Grain-Free

Breakfast: Banana Almond Milk Smoothie with a Scoop of Protein Powder

Lunch: Grilled Salmon with a Side Salad (leafy greens, cucumber, and avocado)

Dinner: Pork Tenderloin with Roasted Root Vegetables (carrots, turnips)

Snacks: Macadamia Nuts; Sliced Radishes

Day 6: Dairy-Free

Breakfast: Scrambled Eggs with Diced Tomato and Spinach

Lunch: Quinoa Bowl with Grilled Vegetables and Hummus

Dinner: Baked Lemon Pepper Chicken with Steamed Broccoli

Snacks: Carrot Sticks; Sunflower Seeds

Day 7: Toxin-Free

Breakfast: Oatmeal with Almond Milk and a Pinch of Nutmeg (ensure gluten-free oats)

Lunch: Baked Cod with a Side of Steamed Mixed Vegetables

Dinner: Vegetable Curry with Cauliflower Rice

Snacks: Pumpkin Seeds; Fresh Veggie Sticks

CHAPTER 6

ADDITIONAL RESOURCES AND SUPPORT

Supplements and Herbal Aids for Hormonal Health

For women over 40, maintaining hormonal balance is not just about dietary changes; supplements and herbal remedies can play a crucial role. As the body ages, it may require additional support to regulate hormone levels effectively. This is where supplements and herbal aids come into play.

Key Supplements for Hormonal Balance:

Vitamin D: Often dubbed the "sunshine vitamin," Vitamin D is crucial for bone health, immune function, and may positively impact hormonal balance.

Omega-3 Fatty Acids: Found in fish oil and flaxseeds, omega-3s are essential for heart health and may help in reducing menstrual pain and balancing mood swings.

Magnesium: This mineral supports hundreds of biochemical reactions in the body, including mood regulation and sleep quality, both of which can influence hormonal health.

Probiotics: Gut health is closely linked to overall health. Probiotics can aid in digestive health, which is essential for proper hormone synthesis and elimination.

B Vitamins: Particularly B6, B12, and folate play a significant role in energy production and can aid in managing symptoms of hormonal fluctuations like fatigue and mood swings.

Herbal Remedies:

Chasteberry (Vitex): Traditionally used to alleviate symptoms of PMS and may help in normalizing menstrual cycles.

Black Cohosh: Often used to manage menopausal symptoms such as hot flashes and night sweats.

Ashwagandha: An adaptogen that can help the body manage stress, which in turn may aid in balancing stress hormones like cortisol.

Maca Root: Known for its potential to boost libido and energy, maca root may also assist in balancing estrogen levels.

Community and Support

Embarking on a hormone reset journey can be challenging, and having a supportive community can make a significant difference. Community support provides emotional encouragement, shared experiences, and practical advice, making the journey less isolating.

Finding Your Community:

Online Forums and Social Media: Platforms like Facebook, Reddit, and specialized health forums can connect you with individuals undergoing similar experiences.

Local Support Groups: Some areas may have local groups that meet regularly. These can be found through community centers, health clinics, or wellness organizations.

Workshops and Seminars: Attending workshops or seminars on hormonal health can provide valuable information and connect you with like-minded individuals.

Building a Support Network:

Family and Friends: Involving close family and friends can provide an immediate support system. Sharing your goals and challenges with them can foster understanding and encouragement.

Healthcare Professionals: Regular consultations with healthcare professionals like nutritionists, endocrinologists, or naturopaths can offer personalized advice and support.

FAQs and Troubleshooting

Embarking on a hormone reset diet can raise numerous questions and sometimes challenges. Addressing these is key to a successful journey.

Common Questions:

How quickly will I see results? The time frame for experiencing changes varies. Some may notice improvements within a few weeks, while for others, it might take longer.

Can I still eat out? Yes, but it requires careful menu selection and potentially requesting modifications to dishes.

What if I have dietary restrictions? The hormone reset diet is flexible and can be adapted to accommodate most dietary restrictions, whether they're based on allergies, intolerances, or personal preferences.

Troubleshooting Tips:

Not Seeing Results: If you're not seeing the desired results, consider revisiting your diet plan with a professional. Hormonal imbalance can be complex, and sometimes slight adjustments are needed.

Dealing with Cravings: Cravings are normal. Finding healthy substitutes and practicing mindful eating can help manage them.

Managing Social Situations: Social events can be challenging when on a specific diet. Planning ahead, bringing your own snacks, or eating beforehand can help.

CONCLUSION

We have explored a comprehensive approach to the Hormone Reset Diet, specifically tailored for women over 40. This diet is designed to address the unique hormonal changes that occur in women during this stage of life, with a focus on improving overall health, metabolism, and well-being through dietary adjustments.

Key Components of the Diet:

Themed Dietary Approaches: We developed a structured meal plan with specific themes for each day of the week, including meatless, sugar-free, fruitless, caffeine-free, grain-free, dairy-free, and toxin-free days. This structure aims to reduce the intake of foods that can negatively impact hormonal balance while promoting a diverse, nutrient-rich diet.

Nutritional Balance: The meal plans provided are rich in vegetables, lean proteins, healthy fats, and other essential nutrients. They are designed to ensure balanced nutrition, focusing on foods that support hormonal health and overall wellness.

Customization and Flexibility: While the meal plans offer a structured approach, they are also flexible enough to accommodate personal dietary needs and preferences. This adaptability is crucial, as individual nutritional requirements can vary widely, especially in the context of hormonal health.

Supplements and Herbal Aids: In addition to dietary changes, we discussed the role of supplements and herbal remedies in supporting hormonal health. Vitamins, minerals, and certain herbs can provide additional support to the body's hormonal systems.

Community and Support: Recognizing the challenges of adopting a new diet, the importance of community support was emphasized. Building a support network, whether through online forums, local groups, or personal connections, can provide valuable encouragement and advice.

Practical Considerations: The meal plans are designed with practicality in mind, incorporating easily accessible ingredients and straightforward recipes. This practical approach is essential for the sustainability of the diet.

FAQs and Troubleshooting: Addressing common questions and concerns is key to ensuring a smooth transition to the hormone reset diet. The provided guidance aims to help individuals navigate potential challenges and make informed decisions about their diet.

The Hormone Reset Diet for Women Over 40 is more than just a dietary plan; it's a holistic approach to improving hormonal balance through nutrition, lifestyle changes, and community support. The detailed meal plans provided serve as a guide to help women navigate the complex interplay between diet and hormonal health. However, it's important to remember that each individual's health journey is unique. Consulting with healthcare professionals for personalized advice and making adjustments to the diet as needed are crucial steps in ensuring the diet's effectiveness and sustainability.

BONUS

Hormone Reset Diet Shopping Guide

Produce

Vegetables: Spinach, kale, broccoli, cauliflower, bell peppers, cucumbers, tomatoes, carrots, asparagus, zucchini, squash, mushrooms, onions, garlic, green beans, Brussels sprouts, lettuce, avocados, sweet potatoes, butternut squash, mixed greens, eggplant, radishes

Fruits (for non-fruitless days): Apples, bananas, mixed berries (strawberries, blueberries, raspberries), lemons, limes

Proteins

Meat & Poultry: Chicken breast, turkey breast, lean ground turkey, pork loin, pork chops, beef (for stir-fry or kebabs)

Fish & Seafood: Salmon, cod, trout, shrimp, tuna (fresh or canned)

Plant-Based Proteins: Tofu, tempeh, lentils, chickpeas, black beans, quinoa, edamame

Dairy & Dairy Alternatives

Dairy: Greek yogurt (plain, unsweetened), eggs, feta cheese (for non-dairy-free days)

Dairy Alternatives: Almond milk, coconut milk, coconut yogurt, dairy-free cheese

Grains & Cereals

Grains (for non-grain-free days): Quinoa, whole grain or gluten-free bread, oatmeal (gluten-free if necessary), brown rice, cauliflower rice

Nuts, Seeds, & Healthy Fats

Nuts & Seeds: Almonds, walnuts, macadamia nuts, pumpkin seeds, sunflower seeds, chia seeds, flaxseeds

Healthy Fats: Olive oil, avocado oil, coconut oil, almond butter

Beverages

Teas: Herbal teas (caffeine-free options)

Others: Almond milk (unsweetened), coconut milk (unsweetened)

Condiments & Spices

Spices: Cinnamon, nutmeg, turmeric, ginger, garlic powder, Italian seasoning, salt, pepper

Condiments: Mustard, vinegar (apple cider, balsamic), low-sodium soy sauce or tamari, lemon juice, tahini

Supplements & Herbal Aids (Optional)

Supplements: Vitamin D, Omega-3 fatty acids, magnesium, probiotics, B vitamins

Herbal Remedies: Chasteberry (Vitex), black cohosh, ashwagandha, maca root

Snacks

Healthy Snacks: Roasted seaweed, hummus, guacamole, unsweetened coconut flakes, boiled eggs, fresh vegetable sticks

www.ingramcontent.com/pod-product-compliance
Lightning Source LLC
Chambersburg PA
CBHW070758260726
48660CB00005B/1681